A MENINGITIS SURVIVAL GUIDE

Understanding the Causes, Symptoms, Diagnosis,Treatment and Prevention Strategies

By

Sherrie A. Jones.

TABLE OF CONTENT

ABOUT THE BOOK

Meningitis is a serious condition characterized by inflammation of the protective membranes covering the brain and spinal cord. It can be caused by a variety of infectious agents, including bacteria, viruses, fungi, and parasites, with bacterial and viral meningitis being the most common forms. While viral meningitis is usually less severe and resolves without specific treatment, bacterial meningitis is a medical emergency that requires prompt diagnosis and treatment to prevent serious complications, including death.

This comprehensive guide aims to provide a detailed overview of meningitis, including its causes, symptoms, diagnosis, treatment, and prevention. We will delve into the different types of meningitis, their respective causes, and the specific diagnostic tests used to identify them. We will also explore the various treatment options available, including antibiotics, antiviral medications, and supportive care.

Additionally, this guide will discuss the importance of vaccination in preventing certain types of meningitis and highlight other preventive measures, such as practicing good hygiene and avoiding close contact with infected individuals. We will also address common misconceptions and provide practical tips for caregivers and individuals recovering from meningitis.

Whether you are a healthcare professional seeking to deepen your understanding of meningitis or an individual looking to protect yourself and your loved ones, this guide is designed to be a valuable resource in unraveling the complexities of this potentially life-threatening disease.

Chapter 1

Introduction to Meningitis

1.1 Definition and Overview

Meningitis is a medical condition characterized by inflammation of the meninges, the protective membranes surrounding the brain and spinal cord. This inflammation is typically caused by an infection, although it can also result from other causes such as medication reactions, cancer, or autoimmune diseases.

The meninges consist of three layers: the dura mater, arachnoid mater, and pia mater. These layers help protect the central nervous system and provide a cushion for the brain and spinal cord.

Meningitis can be classified into several types based on the cause of the infection:

1. **Bacterial Meningitis**: Caused by bacteria such as Streptococcus pneumoniae, Neisseria meningitis, and Haemophilus influenzae. It is a serious and potentially life-threatening condition that requires immediate medical attention.

2. **Viral Meningitis**: Caused by various viruses, including enteroviruses and herpesviruses. Viral meningitis is generally less severe than bacterial meningitis and often resolves on its own without specific treatment.

3. **Fungal Meningitis**: Caused by fungi such as Cryptococcus neoformans. Fungal meningitis is relatively rare but can be serious, especially in individuals with weakened immune systems.

4. **Parasitic Meningitis**: Caused by parasites such as Naegleria fowleri or Trypanosoma brucei. These infections are uncommon but can be life-threatening.

5. **Aseptic Meningitis**: A term used to describe cases of meningitis where no

bacterial or fungal cause is identified. Aseptic meningitis is often caused by viruses and has a better prognosis than bacterial meningitis.

Symptoms of meningitis can vary but often include fever, headache, neck stiffness, and sensitivity to light. In severe cases, it can lead to neurological complications, coma, or death.

Treatment for meningitis depends on the cause and may include antibiotics, antiviral medications, or antifungal drugs. Supportive care, such as pain relief and hydration, is also important for recovery.

Prevention of meningitis can be achieved through vaccination for certain types of bacteria and viruses, practicing good hygiene, and avoiding close contact with infected individuals.

Meningitis is a serious condition that requires prompt diagnosis and treatment. If you suspect you or someone else may have meningitis, seek medical attention immediately.

1.2 Types of Meningitis

Meningitis can be classified into several types based on the cause of the inflammation. The main types of meningitis include bacterial, viral, fungal, parasitic, and aseptic meningitis:

1. **Bacterial Meningitis**: This type of meningitis is caused by bacteria such as Streptococcus pneumoniae, Neisseria meningitidis, and Haemophilus influenzae. Bacterial meningitis is a medical emergency that requires immediate treatment with antibiotics. It can be life-threatening and lead to serious complications if not treated promptly.

2. **Viral Meningitis**: Viral meningitis is caused by various viruses, including enteroviruses, herpesviruses, and others. It is usually less severe than bacterial meningitis and often resolves on its own without specific treatment. However,

supportive care may be needed to manage symptoms.

3. **Fungal Meningitis**: Fungal meningitis is caused by fungi such as Cryptococcus neoformans. It is relatively rare but can be serious, especially in individuals with weakened immune systems. Treatment usually involves antifungal medications.

4. **Parasitic Meningitis**: Parasitic meningitis is caused by parasites such as Naegleria fowleri or Trypanosoma brucei. These infections are uncommon but can be life-threatening. Treatment depends on the specific parasite involved.

5. **Aseptic Meningitis**: Aseptic meningitis is a term used to describe cases of meningitis where no bacterial or fungal cause is identified. It is often caused by viruses and has a better prognosis than bacterial meningitis. Treatment may include supportive care and management of symptoms.

Each type of meningitis has its own causes, symptoms, and treatment options. Proper diagnosis by a healthcare professional is essential to determine the appropriate course of treatment.

1.3 Causes and Risk Factors

Bacterial Meningitis:

- **Causes:** Bacterial meningitis is commonly caused by several types of bacteria, including Streptococcus pneumoniae, Neisseria meningitidis, and Haemophilus influenzae type b (Hib). These bacteria can spread through respiratory droplets or close contact with an infected person.
- **Risk Factors:** Risk factors for bacterial meningitis include age (infants and young children are at higher risk), weakened immune system, living in close quarters (such as college dormitories), and certain

medical conditions (such as a cochlear implant or a history of spleen removal).

2. Viral Meningitis:

- **Causes:** Viral meningitis is most commonly caused by enteroviruses, but other viruses such as herpesviruses, mumps virus, and influenza virus can also cause the infection. These viruses are typically spread through respiratory secretions.
- **Risk Factors:** Risk factors for viral meningitis include age (children under 5 years old are at higher risk), living in crowded conditions, and exposure to someone with a viral infection.

3. Fungal Meningitis:

- **Causes:** Fungal meningitis is caused by various fungi, such as Cryptococcus neoformans. Fungal spores are commonly found in the environment and can be inhaled, leading to infection.

- **Risk Factors:** Risk factors for fungal meningitis include a weakened immune system (such as in HIV/AIDS patients), organ transplantation, and long-term corticosteroid use.

4. Parasitic Meningitis:

- **Causes:** Parasitic meningitis is caused by parasites such as Naegleria fowleri or Trypanosoma brucei. These parasites are typically found in contaminated water sources.
- **Risk Factors:** Risk factors for parasitic meningitis include swimming in warm freshwater lakes and rivers, especially in warm climates.

5. Aseptic Meningitis:

- **Causes:** Aseptic meningitis is often caused by viruses, but it can also be caused by other non-bacterial, non-fungal agents such as medications (e.g.,

nonsteroidal anti-inflammatory drugs, antibiotics) or autoimmune diseases.

- **Risk Factors:** Risk factors for aseptic meningitis depend on the specific cause, but generally include factors that weaken the immune system or increase susceptibility to infections.

6. Non-Infectious Causes:

- Meningitis can also be caused by non-infectious factors such as certain cancers, inflammatory diseases, or reactions to medications.

It's important to note that while certain factors may increase the risk of developing meningitis, anyone can develop the condition. Vaccination and practicing good hygiene can help reduce the risk of bacterial and viral meningitis.

1.4 Signs and Symptoms

The signs and symptoms of meningitis can vary depending on the cause (bacterial, viral, fungal, etc.) and the age of the individual. However, common symptoms include:

1. **Sudden Onset of Fever:** Meningitis often begins with a sudden high fever, which can develop rapidly over a few hours.
2. **Severe Headache:** Individuals with meningitis often experience a severe headache that is different from their usual headaches.
3. **Stiff Neck:** Meningitis can cause a stiff neck, making it difficult to touch your chin to your chest.
4. **Photophobia:** Sensitivity to light is common in meningitis and can cause discomfort in bright light.
5. **Nausea and Vomiting:** Meningitis can cause nausea, vomiting, and in some cases, diarrhea.

6. **Confusion or Altered Mental Status:** Meningitis can lead to confusion, difficulty concentrating, and other mental status changes.
7. **Seizures:** Some individuals with meningitis may experience seizures, especially in severe cases.
8. **Skin Rash:** Certain types of bacterial meningitis, such as meningococcal meningitis, can cause a characteristic skin rash. This rash may appear as small, red or purple spots or bruises.
9. **Other Symptoms:** Other symptoms of meningitis can include lethargy, irritability (especially in infants), joint pain, and muscle aches.

1.5 Diagnosis.

1. **Medical History and Physical Examination:** The healthcare provider will begin by taking a detailed medical

history and conducting a physical examination. They will look for symptoms such as fever, headache, neck stiffness, and altered mental status.

2. **Lumbar Puncture (Spinal Tap):** A lumbar puncture may be performed to collect a sample of cerebrospinal fluid (CSF) for analysis. This test can help identify the presence of bacteria, viruses, or other pathogens in the CSF.

3. **CSF Analysis:** The collected CSF sample will be analyzed for cell count, glucose level, protein level, and presence of bacteria or viruses. Abnormalities in these parameters can indicate meningitis.

4. **Blood Tests:** Blood tests may be conducted to check for signs of infection, such as elevated white blood cell count and inflammatory markers.

5. **Imaging Studies:** In some cases, imaging studies such as a CT scan or MRI may be performed to look for signs of

inflammation or other abnormalities in the brain and spinal cord.

6. **Viral Testing:** If viral meningitis is suspected, additional tests may be performed to identify the specific virus causing the infection.

7. **Other Tests:** Depending on the suspected cause of meningitis, additional tests such as PCR (polymerase chain reaction) testing, serologic tests, or cultures may be conducted to identify the pathogen.

8. **Differential Diagnosis:** Meningitis can have symptoms similar to other conditions, so the healthcare provider will consider other possible causes of symptoms and may perform additional tests to rule out other conditions.

9. **Clinical Presentation:** The healthcare provider will also consider the overall clinical presentation of the patient, including symptoms, medical history, and physical examination findings, to make a diagnosis.

Chapter 2

Understanding the Meninges and Central Nervous System

2.1 Anatomy of the Meninges

The meninges are three layers of protective membranes that surround the brain and spinal cord. These layers provide a barrier between the central nervous system (CNS) structures and the surrounding skull and vertebrae. Here's an overview of the anatomy of the meninges:

1. **Dura Mater:** The outermost layer of the meninges is the dura mater, which is a tough, fibrous membrane. It serves as a protective barrier and helps support the brain and spinal cord. The dura mater is attached to the inner surface of the skull and extends into the vertebral canal.

2. **Arachnoid Mater:** The middle layer of the meninges is the arachnoid mater, which is a thin, web-like membrane. The space between the arachnoid mater and the pia mater is called the subarachnoid space, which contains cerebrospinal fluid (CSF) that helps cushion the brain and spinal cord.

3. **Pia Mater:** The innermost layer of the meninges is the pia mater, which is a thin, delicate membrane that closely covers the surface of the brain and spinal cord. It contains blood vessels that supply nutrients and oxygen to the CNS structures.

The meninges help protect the brain and spinal cord from injury and infection. They also play a role in maintaining the environment surrounding the CNS, including regulating the flow of CSF. Disorders affecting the meninges, such as meningitis, can lead to serious health problems and require prompt medical attention.

2.2 Role of the Central Nervous System

The central nervous system (CNS) is directly affected by meningitis, as the disease involves inflammation of the meninges, the protective membranes surrounding the brain and spinal cord. Here's how the CNS is involved in meningitis:

1. **Inflammation and Immune Response:** Meningitis is typically caused by an infection, either bacterial, viral, fungal, or parasitic. When pathogens enter the CNS, the immune system responds by triggering inflammation in an attempt to fight off the infection. This inflammation can cause damage to the meninges and surrounding tissues.

2. **Increased Intracranial Pressure:** Inflammation in the subarachnoid space

(the space between the arachnoid mater and pia mater, which contains cerebrospinal fluid) can lead to increased intracranial pressure. This pressure can compress the brain and interfere with its normal functioning.

3. **Symptoms and Neurological Effects:** The inflammation and increased pressure associated with meningitis can lead to a variety of symptoms, including headache, neck stiffness, photophobia, altered mental status, and seizures. These symptoms are the result of the CNS being affected by the inflammatory process.

4. **Complications:** Meningitis can lead to serious complications affecting the CNS, such as hydrocephalus (accumulation of fluid in the brain), brain abscesses, cranial nerve palsies, and neurological deficits. These complications can result from direct damage caused by the infection or from the body's immune response to the infection.

5. **Treatment and Management:** Treatment of meningitis often involves antibiotics or antiviral medications to combat the infection. Corticosteroids may also be used to reduce inflammation. Supportive care, including management of intracranial pressure and neurological symptoms, is important for a successful outcome.

Chapter 3

Bacterial Meningitis

3.1 Causes and Pathogenesis

Bacterial meningitis is primarily caused by several types of bacteria, including Streptococcus pneumoniae, Neisseria meningitidis, and Haemophilus influenzae type b (Hib). These bacteria can enter the body through the respiratory tract or bloodstream and then spread to the meninges, leading to inflammation and infection. The pathogenesis of bacterial meningitis involves several key steps:

1. **Transmission:** Bacterial meningitis is typically transmitted through respiratory droplets or direct contact with respiratory secretions from an infected person. Close contact, such as living in close quarters or

sharing utensils, can increase the risk of transmission.

2. **Invasion:** Once the bacteria enter the body, they can invade the bloodstream and cross the blood-brain barrier to reach the meninges. Certain factors, such as virulence factors produced by the bacteria, can enhance their ability to invade and survive in the CNS.

3. **Inflammation:** The presence of bacteria in the meninges triggers an immune response, leading to inflammation. This inflammatory response is characterized by the release of cytokines, chemokines, and other inflammatory mediators, which can cause damage to the meninges and surrounding tissues.

4. **Symptoms:** The inflammatory response in bacterial meningitis results in symptoms such as fever, headache, neck stiffness, and altered mental status. These symptoms are the body's natural response to the infection and inflammation.

5. **Complications:** Bacterial meningitis can lead to serious complications, including brain damage, hearing loss, seizures, and death. These complications can result from the direct effects of the infection on the brain and surrounding tissues, as well as from the body's immune response to the infection.

6. **Treatment:** Treatment of bacterial meningitis typically involves antibiotics to eradicate the bacteria. Corticosteroids may also be used to reduce inflammation. Prompt diagnosis and treatment are crucial to reduce the risk of complications and improve outcomes.

7. **Prevention:** Vaccination is an important preventive measure against bacterial meningitis. Vaccines are available for certain types of bacteria that commonly cause meningitis, such as pneumococcal, meningococcal, and Hib vaccines. Maintaining good hygiene practices, such as washing hands regularly and avoiding

close contact with infected individuals, can also help prevent the spread of bacteria that cause meningitis.

3.2 Clinical Presentation

The clinical presentation of bacterial meningitis can vary depending on the age of the patient, the specific bacteria causing the infection, and the severity of the illness. However, there are several common symptoms and signs that are often seen in cases of bacterial meningitis:

1. **Sudden Onset of Fever:** Bacterial meningitis often begins with a sudden high fever, which can develop rapidly over a few hours.
2. **Severe Headache:** Individuals with bacterial meningitis typically experience a severe headache that is different from their usual headaches.
3. **Stiff Neck:** Meningitis can cause a stiff neck, making it difficult to touch your

chin to your chest. This is known as nuchal rigidity.

4. **Photophobia:** Sensitivity to light is common in bacterial meningitis and can cause discomfort in bright light.

5. **Nausea and Vomiting:** Bacterial meningitis can cause nausea, vomiting, and in some cases, diarrhea.

6. **Altered Mental Status:** Bacterial meningitis can lead to confusion, difficulty concentrating, and other mental status changes.

7. **Seizures:** Some individuals with bacterial meningitis may experience seizures, especially in severe cases.

8. **Skin Rash:** Certain types of bacterial meningitis, such as meningococcal meningitis, can cause a characteristic skin rash. This rash may appear as small, red or purple spots or bruises.

9. **Other Symptoms:** Other symptoms of bacterial meningitis can include lethargy,

irritability (especially in infants), joint pain, and muscle aches.

3.3 Diagnostic Approach

The diagnostic approach to bacterial meningitis involves a combination of medical history, physical examination, laboratory tests, and imaging studies. Here's an overview of the diagnostic process:

1. **Medical History:** The healthcare provider will ask about symptoms, recent illnesses, and any recent exposure to individuals with meningitis or other infections.
2. **Physical Examination:** The healthcare provider will perform a thorough physical examination, focusing on signs of meningitis such as fever, neck stiffness, and neurological deficits.
3. **Lumbar Puncture (Spinal Tap):** A lumbar puncture may be performed to

collect a sample of cerebrospinal fluid (CSF) for analysis. This test is essential for diagnosing meningitis and determining the specific cause (bacterial, viral, fungal, etc.). In bacterial meningitis, the CSF often shows increased white blood cell count, elevated protein levels, and decreased glucose levels.

4. **CSF Analysis:** The collected CSF sample is analyzed for cell count, glucose level, protein level, and presence of bacteria or viruses. Gram staining and culture of the CSF can help identify the specific bacteria causing the infection.

5. **Blood Tests:** Blood tests may be conducted to check for signs of infection, such as elevated white blood cell count and inflammatory markers.

6. **Imaging Studies:** Imaging studies such as a CT scan or MRI may be performed to look for signs of inflammation or other abnormalities in the brain and spinal cord. These imaging studies can help rule out

other conditions and assess for complications of meningitis.

7. **Other Tests:** Depending on the suspected cause of meningitis, additional tests such as PCR (polymerase chain reaction) testing, serologic tests, or cultures may be conducted to identify the pathogen.

8. **Differential Diagnosis:** Meningitis can have symptoms similar to other conditions, so the healthcare provider will consider other possible causes of symptoms and may perform additional tests to rule out other conditions.

9. **Clinical Presentation:** The healthcare provider will also consider the overall clinical presentation of the patient, including symptoms, medical history, and physical examination findings, to make a diagnosis.

3.4 Treatment and Management

Treatment and management of bacterial meningitis typically involve a combination of antibiotics, supportive care, and monitoring for complications. Here's an overview of the treatment approach:

1. **Antibiotics:** Bacterial meningitis is treated with antibiotics, usually given intravenously. The choice of antibiotic depends on the specific bacteria causing the infection, as well as local antibiotic resistance patterns. Commonly used antibiotics include third-generation cephalosporins (e.g., ceftriaxone or cefotaxime) and vancomycin.

2. **Corticosteroids:** In some cases, corticosteroids such as dexamethasone may be used in conjunction with antibiotics to reduce inflammation in the brain and improve outcomes. Corticosteroids are typically used in cases of suspected or confirmed bacterial

meningitis caused by Streptococcus pneumoniae.

3. **Supportive Care:** Supportive care is important for managing symptoms and complications of bacterial meningitis. This may include pain management, fever reduction, and management of dehydration and electrolyte imbalances.

4. **Monitoring:** Patients with bacterial meningitis require close monitoring for signs of improvement or deterioration. This may include regular assessment of vital signs, neurological status, and laboratory parameters such as CSF analysis.

5. **Seizure Management:** Patients with bacterial meningitis are at increased risk of seizures, so seizure precautions and management may be necessary.

6. **Isolation Precautions:** Bacterial meningitis is contagious, so isolation precautions may be necessary to prevent

the spread of infection, especially in healthcare settings.

7. **Treatment of Complications:** Bacterial meningitis can lead to serious complications such as brain damage, hearing loss, and neurological deficits. These complications may require additional treatment and rehabilitation.

8. **Follow-Up:** Patients recovering from bacterial meningitis may require follow-up care to monitor for long-term complications and ensure complete recovery.

9. **Prevention:** Vaccination is an important preventive measure against bacterial meningitis. Vaccines are available for certain types of bacteria that commonly cause meningitis, such as pneumococcal, meningococcal, and Hib vaccines.

3.5 Prevention Strategies

1. **Vaccination**: Vaccines are available for certain types of bacterial meningitis, such as those caused by Neisseria meningitidis, Streptococcus pneumoniae, and Haemophilus influenzae type b (Hib). Getting vaccinated according to the recommended schedule can help prevent these types of meningitis.

2. **Good Hygiene**: Practicing good hygiene, such as washing hands frequently and avoiding sharing utensils or personal items, can help prevent the spread of viruses and bacteria that can cause meningitis.

3. **Avoiding Close Contact**: Avoiding close contact with individuals who have viral or bacterial infections that can lead to meningitis can reduce the risk of transmission.

4. **Maintaining a Healthy Lifestyle**: A healthy lifestyle, including getting enough

rest, eating a balanced diet, and managing stress, can help support a strong immune system, which may reduce the risk of infections that can lead to meningitis.

5. **Prompt Treatment of Infections**: Treating infections that can lead to meningitis, such as ear infections or pneumonia, promptly and effectively can help prevent them from progressing to meningitis.

6. **Chemoprophylaxis**: In certain situations, such as when someone has been in close contact with a person diagnosed with bacterial meningitis, doctors may recommend antibiotics to prevent the infection from spreading.

Chapter 4

Viral Meningitis

4.1 Etiology and Transmission

Bacterial Meningitis:

- Common bacteria causing bacterial meningitis include Streptococcus pneumoniae, Neisseria meningitidis, and Haemophilus influenzae type b (Hib).
- Transmission often occurs through respiratory droplets from coughs or sneezes of an infected person. It can also spread through close contact, such as kissing, or sharing items like eating utensils or toothbrushes.

Viral Meningitis:

- Viral meningitis is most often caused by enteroviruses, but other viruses such as herpes simplex virus, mumps virus, and West Nile virus can also lead to viral meningitis.
- Transmission typically occurs through contact with respiratory secretions (saliva, sputum, or nasal mucus) or fecal contamination.

Fungal Meningitis:

- Fungal meningitis is usually caused by inhaling fungal spores from the environment. Cryptococcus neoformans is a common fungal cause of meningitis, especially in people with weakened immune systems.

Parasitic Meningitis:

- Parasitic meningitis is rare but can occur due to parasites such as Naegleria fowleri, which is found in warm freshwater environments. Infection usually occurs when contaminated water enters the body through the nose.

Non-Infectious Causes:

- Meningitis can also be caused by non-infectious factors such as certain medications, autoimmune diseases, cancer, and some inflammatory conditions.

4.2 Clinical Features

The clinical features of meningitis can vary depending on the cause (bacterial, viral, fungal, etc.) and the age and overall health of the individual. However, some common symptoms and signs include:

1. **Fever**: A high fever is often present, especially in bacterial meningitis.
2. **Headache**: Severe, persistent headache is a common symptom of meningitis.

3. **Stiff Neck**: Neck stiffness, especially when trying to touch the chin to the chest, is a classic symptom.
4. **Photophobia**: Sensitivity to light is common in meningitis.
5. **Altered Mental Status**: Confusion, irritability, or changes in behavior can occur, especially in severe cases.
6. **Nausea and Vomiting**: These symptoms are common, particularly in the early stages of the illness.
7. **Seizures**: Seizures can occur in some cases, especially in bacterial meningitis.
8. **Skin Rash**: In meningococcal meningitis, a characteristic rash may develop. The rash may be small, red or purple spots or larger bruises.
9. **In infants**: Symptoms can be less specific and may include irritability, poor feeding, and a bulging fontanelle (soft spot on the baby's head).

4.3 Diagnosis and Differential Diagnosis

Diagnosing meningitis typically involves a combination of clinical evaluation, laboratory tests, and imaging studies. The process may include the following steps:

1. **Medical History and Physical Examination**: The healthcare provider will review the patient's symptoms and perform a physical exam, focusing on signs of meningitis such as neck stiffness, altered mental status, and skin rash.

2. **Lumbar Puncture (Spinal Tap)**: This is a key diagnostic test for meningitis. A sample of cerebrospinal fluid (CSF) is collected through a needle inserted into the lower back. The CSF is then tested for signs of infection, such as an elevated white blood cell count and the presence of bacteria, viruses, or other pathogens.

3. **Blood Tests**: Blood tests can help identify the cause of meningitis by detecting signs of infection, such as elevated white blood cell count or specific antibodies.

4. **Imaging Studies**: In some cases, imaging studies such as CT scans or MRI scans may be performed to look for signs of inflammation or other abnormalities in the brain and surrounding structures.

5. **Microbiological Tests**: If bacterial or fungal meningitis is suspected, microbiological tests may be performed on CSF or blood samples to identify the specific organism causing the infection.

Differential Diagnosis:

- **Viral Meningitis**: This is the most common type of meningitis and is often less severe than bacterial meningitis. It can be challenging to distinguish from bacterial meningitis based solely on symptoms, so laboratory tests are essential for accurate diagnosis.

- **Fungal Meningitis**: This type of meningitis is less common and often occurs in people with weakened immune systems. Diagnosis is made based on CSF analysis and sometimes requires specialized tests.
- **Non-Infectious Causes**: Conditions such as autoimmune disorders, certain medications, and some cancers can mimic the symptoms of meningitis. A thorough medical history, physical exam, and diagnostic tests are crucial for identifying these causes.

4.4 Management and Prognosis

Management of meningitis involves treating the underlying cause and providing supportive care to manage symptoms and prevent complications. The specific approach depends on the type of meningitis (bacterial, viral, fungal, etc.) and the severity of the infection. Here are some general strategies:

1. **Antibiotics or Antiviral Medications**: For bacterial meningitis, antibiotics are usually started immediately, often intravenously, based on the likely causative organism until specific information from cultures is available. Viral meningitis typically does not respond to antibiotics, so antiviral medications may be used if the cause is suspected to be viral.
2. **Antifungal Medications**: Fungal meningitis requires treatment with antifungal medications, which may need to be taken for an extended period.
3. **Supportive Care**: Supportive measures such as pain relief, fever control, and hydration are important. In severe cases, patients may require hospitalization and supportive treatments such as oxygen therapy or mechanical ventilation.

4. **Monitoring and Complication Management**: Patients with meningitis need close monitoring for complications such as seizures, increased intracranial pressure, and neurological deficits. These complications may require specific treatments.

5. **Preventive Measures**: Depending on the type of meningitis, preventive measures such as vaccination (for bacterial and viral meningitis), avoiding mosquito bites (for some types of viral meningitis), and practicing good hygiene can help prevent meningitis.

Prognosis:

- **Bacterial Meningitis**: This can be life-threatening, especially if not treated promptly. However, with appropriate antibiotics, most people recover completely. Some may have long-term complications such as hearing loss, cognitive deficits, or seizures.

- **Viral Meningitis**: Most cases are mild and resolve on their own without specific treatment. The prognosis is generally good, with full recovery expected in the majority of cases.
- **Fungal Meningitis**: This type of meningitis can be more challenging to treat, especially in people with weakened immune systems. The prognosis depends on the underlying cause and the effectiveness of antifungal therapy.
- **Non-Infectious Meningitis**: The prognosis depends on the underlying cause. With appropriate management, outcomes can vary widely.

Chapter 5

Fungal and Parasitic Meningitis

5.1 Overview of Fungal Meningitis

Fungal meningitis is a rare but serious condition caused by fungal infection of the membranes (meninges) surrounding the brain and spinal cord. Unlike bacterial and viral meningitis, which are more common, fungal meningitis is usually not contagious.

Causes: Fungal meningitis can be caused by several types of fungi. The most common causes include Cryptococcus, Histoplasma, and Coccidioides species. These fungi are typically found in the environment, particularly in soil contaminated with bird droppings

(Cryptococcus) or in areas with high concentrations of bat or bird droppings (Histoplasma and Coccidioides).

Risk Factors: Individuals with weakened immune systems are at higher risk of developing fungal meningitis. This includes people with HIV/AIDS, those taking medications that suppress the immune system (such as corticosteroids or chemotherapy), and individuals with certain underlying medical conditions.

Symptoms: The symptoms of fungal meningitis are similar to those of other types of meningitis and can include fever, headache, stiff neck, nausea, vomiting, sensitivity to light, and altered mental status.

Diagnosis: Diagnosis is made through a combination of clinical evaluation, imaging studies (such as CT or MRI scans), and laboratory tests. A lumbar puncture (spinal tap) is typically performed to collect cerebrospinal fluid (CSF) for analysis.

Treatment: Fungal meningitis is treated with antifungal medications, which may need to be given intravenously for an extended period. The specific antifungal medication and duration of treatment depend on the type of fungus causing the infection and the severity of the illness.

Prognosis: The prognosis for fungal meningitis varies depending on the type of fungus causing the infection, the underlying health of the individual, and how quickly the infection is diagnosed and treated. In general, early and aggressive treatment can lead to a good outcome, but the condition can be life-threatening if not treated promptly.

Prevention: Preventive measures for fungal meningitis include avoiding areas with high concentrations of bird or bat droppings, especially for individuals with weakened immune systems. In some cases, antifungal medications may be used prophylactically in high-risk individuals.

5.2 Overview of Parasitic Meningitis

Parasitic meningitis is a rare but serious condition caused by parasitic infections that affect the membranes (meninges) surrounding the brain and spinal cord. The two most common types of parasitic meningitis are caused by the amoeba Naegleria fowleri and the roundworm Angiostrongylus cantonensis.

1. Naegleria fowleri Meningoencephalitis:

- **Cause:** Naegleria fowleri is found in warm freshwater environments, such as lakes, rivers, and hot springs. Infection occurs when contaminated water enters the body through the nose.

- **Symptoms:** Initial symptoms can resemble bacterial meningitis and include headache, fever, nausea, and vomiting. As the infection progresses, symptoms may worsen to include stiff neck, confusion, seizures, and hallucinations.
- **Diagnosis:** Diagnosis is made by detecting the parasite in cerebrospinal fluid (CSF) obtained through a lumbar puncture (spinal tap).
- **Treatment:** Treatment is challenging, and medications such as amphotericin B and miltefosine, along with supportive care, may be used. However, the infection is often fatal.

2. *Angiostrongylus cantonensis* Meningoencephalitis:

- **Cause:** Angiostrongylus cantonensis is a parasitic roundworm found in rats, which can be transmitted to humans through consumption of contaminated food, particularly raw or undercooked snails and slugs.

- **Symptoms:** Symptoms can vary but often include headache, neck stiffness, fever, nausea, and vomiting. In severe cases, neurological symptoms such as weakness, paralysis, and coma may occur.
- **Diagnosis:** Diagnosis is made based on clinical symptoms, exposure history, and sometimes by detecting the parasite in CSF.
- **Treatment:** Treatment may involve medications to reduce inflammation and swelling in the brain, along with supportive care. In some cases, antiparasitic medications may be used.

Prevention: Preventive measures include avoiding swimming or diving in warm freshwater where Naegleria fowleri may be present, and ensuring food hygiene to prevent Angiostrongylus cantonensis infection.

5.3 Diagnosis and Treatment

Diagnosis of parasitic meningitis involves a combination of clinical evaluation, laboratory tests, and sometimes imaging studies. The specific approach may vary depending on the suspected parasite causing the infection. Here is an overview:

Diagnosis:

1. **Clinical Evaluation:** Symptoms such as headache, fever, stiff neck, and neurological signs may raise suspicion of meningitis. A detailed medical history, including recent travel or exposure to potential sources of infection, is important.
2. **Laboratory Tests:**
    - **Cerebrospinal Fluid (CSF) Analysis:** A lumbar puncture (spinal tap) is performed to collect CSF for analysis. This can help identify the presence of parasites,

white blood cell count (indicating inflammation), and other markers of infection.

- **Microscopic Examination:** The CSF sample is examined under a microscope to look for parasites or their eggs (larvae) that may be causing the infection.

- **Other Tests:** Depending on the suspected parasite, additional tests may be performed, such as serological tests or polymerase chain reaction (PCR) tests to detect specific parasite DNA.

3. **Imaging Studies:** CT scans or MRI scans of the brain may be done to look for signs of inflammation, swelling, or other abnormalities.

Treatment:

1. **Antiparasitic Medications:** Treatment typically involves antiparasitic medications specific to the parasite

causing the infection. Examples include amphotericin B or miltefosine for Naegleria fowleri infection and albendazole or mebendazole for Angiostrongylus cantonensis infection.

2. **Supportive Care:** Supportive measures may include medications to reduce fever, pain, and inflammation, as well as management of complications such as seizures or increased intracranial pressure.

3. **Hospitalization:** Severe cases of parasitic meningitis may require hospitalization for close monitoring and management.

4. **Follow-Up:** Regular follow-up with healthcare providers is important to monitor the response to treatment and manage any long-term effects or complications.

Chapter 6

Aseptic Meningitis

6.1 Definition and Causes

Aseptic meningitis, also known as viral meningitis, is a condition characterized by inflammation of the membranes (meninges) surrounding the brain and spinal cord. Unlike bacterial meningitis, which is caused by bacterial infection, aseptic meningitis is typically caused by viral infections. However, other non-bacterial causes such as certain medications, autoimmune disorders, and fungal infections can also lead to aseptic meningitis.

Causes:

1. **Viruses:** The most common cause of aseptic meningitis is viral infections. Enteroviruses, including coxsackievirus

and echovirus, are the most frequent culprits. Other viruses such as herpes simplex virus, varicella-zoster virus (which causes chickenpox and shingles), and mumps virus can also cause aseptic meningitis.

2. **Other Infectious Agents:** Besides viruses, other infectious agents such as fungi (e.g., Cryptococcus neoformans) and parasites (e.g., Angiostrongylus cantonensis) can also lead to aseptic meningitis, although these are less common causes.

3. **Non-Infectious Causes:** Aseptic meningitis can also be caused by non-infectious factors, including certain medications (e.g., nonsteroidal anti-inflammatory drugs, antibiotics, intravenous immunoglobulin), autoimmune disorders (e.g., systemic lupus erythematosus, sarcoidosis), and some cancers.

Risk Factors:

- Individuals of all ages can develop aseptic meningitis, but certain factors may increase the risk. These include being younger than 30 years old, living in crowded conditions, having a weakened immune system, and recent exposure to someone with viral meningitis.

Transmission:

- Viral meningitis is typically spread through close contact with an infected person, exposure to respiratory droplets from coughs or sneezes, or contact with contaminated surfaces. Non-viral causes of aseptic meningitis are not contagious.

Aseptic meningitis often presents with symptoms similar to bacterial meningitis, such as fever, headache, stiff neck, nausea, vomiting, sensitivity to light (photophobia), and altered mental status. However, the course of the illness and the severity of symptoms are generally milder in aseptic meningitis compared to bacterial meningitis.

6.2 Clinical Presentation

The clinical presentation of aseptic meningitis can vary depending on the underlying cause and the age and overall health of the individual. However, there are some common signs and symptoms to be aware of:

1. **Fever:** A high fever is often present, usually over 100.4°F (38°C).
2. **Headache:** Severe, persistent headache is a common symptom of meningitis.
3. **Stiff Neck:** Neck stiffness, especially when trying to touch the chin to the chest, is a classic symptom.
4. **Photophobia:** Sensitivity to light is common in meningitis.

5. **Altered Mental Status:** Confusion, irritability, or changes in behavior can occur, especially in severe cases.

6. **Nausea and Vomiting:** These symptoms are common, particularly in the early stages of the illness.

7. **Other Symptoms:** Other symptoms may include fatigue, muscle aches, rash, and sore throat, depending on the underlying cause of the meningitis.

It's important to note that not everyone with aseptic meningitis will have all of these symptoms, and symptoms can vary in severity. In some cases, especially in young children or older adults, the symptoms may be less specific or more subtle. Prompt medical evaluation is crucial if meningitis is suspected, as early diagnosis and treatment can help prevent complications.

6.3 Diagnosis and Management

1. **Medical History and Physical Examination:** The healthcare provider will ask about symptoms and perform a physical exam, focusing on signs of meningitis such as neck stiffness, altered mental status, and skin rash.

2. **Lumbar Puncture (Spinal Tap):** This is a key diagnostic test for meningitis. A sample of cerebrospinal fluid (CSF) is collected through a needle inserted into the lower back. The CSF is then tested for signs of infection, such as an elevated white blood cell count and the presence of viruses or other pathogens.

3. **Laboratory Tests:** Blood tests may be done to check for signs of infection or inflammation. Viral cultures, polymerase chain reaction (PCR) tests, or other specialized tests may be performed on CSF to identify the specific virus causing the infection.

4. **Imaging Studies:** In some cases, imaging studies such as CT scans or MRI scans may be performed to look for signs of inflammation or other abnormalities in the brain and surrounding structures.

Management of Aseptic Meningitis:

1. **Supportive Care:** Most cases of aseptic meningitis resolve on their own without specific treatment. Supportive care may include rest, hydration, and over-the-counter pain relievers to help alleviate symptoms such as fever and headache.
2. **Antiviral Medications:** If the cause of aseptic meningitis is a viral infection, antiviral medications may be prescribed in some cases.
3. **Hospitalization:** Severe cases of aseptic meningitis or cases in individuals with weakened immune systems may require hospitalization for close monitoring and supportive care.

4. **Follow-Up:** Regular follow-up with healthcare providers is important to monitor the progress of the illness and ensure that it is resolving appropriately.

Chapter 7

Neonatal Meningitis

7.1 Risk Factors and Etiology

Neonatal meningitis is a serious condition that affects infants less than 1 month old. It can be caused by bacteria, viruses, or, less commonly, fungi. Early recognition and treatment are crucial for a positive outcome.

Risk Factors:

1. **Age:** Neonates are at higher risk due to their immature immune systems.
2. **Prematurity:** Preterm infants are more vulnerable.
3. **Maternal Factors:** Maternal infection during pregnancy can increase the risk.

4. **Delivery:** Prolonged rupture of membranes or invasive procedures during delivery can introduce pathogens.
5. **Low Birth Weight:** Infants with low birth weight are at increased risk.
6. **Invasive Procedures:** Procedures like lumbar punctures or intravascular catheterization can introduce pathogens.
7. **NICU Stay:** Infants in the neonatal intensive care unit (NICU) are at higher risk due to increased exposure to pathogens.

Etiology:

1. **Bacterial:** The most common bacteria causing neonatal meningitis are Group B Streptococcus (GBS), Escherichia coli (E. coli), and Listeria monocytogenes.
2. **Viral:** Viruses such as herpes simplex virus (HSV) and enteroviruses can also cause neonatal meningitis.

3. **Fungal:** Fungal infections, though rare, can occur, typically caused by Candida species.

Transmission: Neonatal meningitis can occur through vertical transmission from the mother during childbirth, postnatal transmission through contact with infected individuals, or nosocomial transmission in healthcare settings.

Clinical Presentation: Symptoms can include fever, lethargy, poor feeding, irritability, seizures, bulging fontanelle, and respiratory distress.

Diagnosis: Diagnosis involves clinical evaluation, blood tests, imaging studies (such as ultrasound or MRI), and analysis of cerebrospinal fluid (CSF) obtained through a lumbar puncture.

Treatment: Treatment typically involves hospitalization and intravenous antibiotics or antiviral medications, depending on the suspected cause. Supportive care to manage symptoms and complications is also important.

Prognosis: The prognosis for neonatal meningitis depends on various factors, including the causative organism, the promptness of treatment, and the presence of any complications. Early diagnosis and treatment can improve outcomes.

7.2 Clinical Presentation in Neonates

Neonatal meningitis can present with a variety of symptoms, but the signs may be subtle and nonspecific, especially in the early stages. The clinical presentation can vary depending on the age of the infant, the causative organism, and other factors. Common symptoms and signs include:

1. **Fever:** Neonates with meningitis often present with fever, although some infants may have low body temperature (hypothermia) instead.
2. **Irritability or Lethargy:** Infants may be irritable, fussy, or difficult to console, or they may appear unusually sleepy or lethargic.
3. **Poor Feeding:** Infants with meningitis may feed poorly or refuse to feed altogether.
4. **Vomiting or Poor Weight Gain:** Some infants may experience vomiting, which can contribute to poor weight gain.
5. **Bulging Fontanelle:** The fontanelle (soft spot on the baby's head) may appear swollen or bulging, although this is not always present.
6. **Seizures:** Neonatal meningitis can cause seizures, which may be subtle and difficult to detect in young infants.

7. **Respiratory Distress:** Some infants may have difficulty breathing or exhibit signs of respiratory distress.

8. **Jaundice:** In some cases, neonatal meningitis may be associated with jaundice (yellowing of the skin and eyes).

9. **Hypotonia or Rigidity:** Infants with meningitis may have abnormal muscle tone, which can manifest as either floppy (hypotonic) or stiff (rigid) muscles.

10. **Other Signs:** Other signs of neonatal meningitis can include a high-pitched cry, irritability when handled, and a general appearance of being unwell.

7.3 Diagnosis and Management

Diagnosis:

1. **Clinical Evaluation:** The healthcare provider will assess the infant's symptoms, medical history, and perform a

physical examination, focusing on signs of meningitis such as fever, irritability, lethargy, and poor feeding.

2. **Laboratory Tests:**
   - **Cerebrospinal Fluid (CSF) Analysis:** A lumbar puncture (spinal tap) is performed to collect CSF for analysis. CSF analysis can reveal an elevated white blood cell count, elevated protein levels, and the presence of bacteria or other pathogens.
   - **Blood Cultures:** Blood samples may be taken to check for the presence of bacteria or other pathogens in the bloodstream.
   - **Other Tests:** Depending on the suspected cause of meningitis, additional tests such as viral PCR, bacterial antigen testing, or fungal cultures may be performed.

3. **Imaging Studies:** Imaging studies such as ultrasound, CT scan, or MRI may be done

to look for signs of inflammation or other abnormalities in the brain.

Management:

1. **Antibiotic or Antiviral Therapy:** Empirical antibiotic therapy is usually initiated immediately after obtaining blood and CSF samples for culture. The choice of antibiotics depends on the likely causative organisms and local resistance patterns. Antiviral therapy may be considered for viral meningitis.
2. **Supportive Care:** Supportive measures may include intravenous fluids, oxygen therapy, and medications to reduce fever and manage seizures.
3. **Monitoring:** Infants with meningitis require close monitoring of vital signs, neurologic status, and response to treatment.
4. **Complications:** Complications of neonatal meningitis may include hydrocephalus, brain abscess, hearing

loss, developmental delays, and long-term neurologic deficits. These infants may require ongoing monitoring and management of complications.

5. **Follow-Up:** Regular follow-up with healthcare providers is important to monitor the infant's progress and ensure appropriate treatment.

Prevention:

- **Maternal Screening and Prophylaxis:** Screening for Group B Streptococcus (GBS) during pregnancy and administering intrapartum antibiotics to GBS-positive mothers can help prevent early-onset neonatal meningitis.
- **Vaccination:** Vaccination of pregnant women against influenza and pertussis can help prevent infections that can lead to neonatal meningitis.
- **Hand Hygiene and Infection Control:** Proper hand hygiene and infection control measures in healthcare settings can help

prevent the spread of infections that can cause neonatal meningitis.

Chapter 8

Meningitis in Special Populations

8.1 Meningitis in Children

Meningitis in children is a serious condition characterized by inflammation of the membranes (meninges) surrounding the brain and spinal cord. It can be caused by bacteria, viruses, fungi, or other pathogens. Prompt diagnosis and treatment are essential to prevent complications and improve outcomes. Here's an overview:

Causes:

1. **Bacterial Meningitis:** Common bacterial causes include Streptococcus pneumoniae, Neisseria meningitidis, and Haemophilus influenzae type b (Hib). Bacterial

meningitis is more severe and requires urgent treatment.

2. **Viral Meningitis:** Viruses such as enteroviruses, herpes simplex virus (HSV), and varicella-zoster virus (VZV) are common causes of viral meningitis. Viral meningitis is generally less severe than bacterial meningitis.

3. **Fungal Meningitis:** Fungal infections, although rare, can also cause meningitis, especially in children with compromised immune systems.

Risk Factors:

- Age: Children under 5 years old, especially infants, are at higher risk.
- Daycare Attendance: Children in daycare settings may have increased exposure to pathogens.
- Immunocompromised State: Children with weakened immune systems are more susceptible to infections.

- Lack of Vaccination: Some vaccine-preventable diseases can cause meningitis if left unvaccinated.

Clinical Presentation:

- Symptoms can vary but often include fever, headache, stiff neck, nausea, vomiting, sensitivity to light (photophobia), and altered mental status. In infants, symptoms may be more subtle and may include irritability, poor feeding, and a bulging fontanelle.

Diagnosis:

- Clinical Evaluation: The healthcare provider will assess the child's symptoms, medical history, and perform a physical exam.
- Lumbar Puncture: A sample of cerebrospinal fluid (CSF) is collected through a lumbar puncture and tested for signs of infection.

- Blood Tests: Blood tests may be done to check for signs of infection and inflammation.

Treatment:

- Bacterial Meningitis: Requires urgent treatment with antibiotics. The choice of antibiotics depends on the likely causative organism and local resistance patterns.
- Viral Meningitis: Generally does not require specific treatment and often resolves on its own. Supportive care is provided to manage symptoms.
- Fungal Meningitis: Treated with antifungal medications, which may need to be given for an extended period.

Prevention:

- Vaccination: Vaccination is the most effective way to prevent many types of bacterial meningitis. Vaccines against Hib, pneumococcus, and meningococcus are recommended for children.

- Hygiene: Practicing good hygiene, such as washing hands regularly, can help prevent the spread of infections that can cause meningitis.

8.2 Meningitis in the Elderly

Meningitis in the elderly is a serious condition that can have significant morbidity and mortality rates. The presentation, diagnosis, and management of meningitis in older adults can differ from that in younger populations. Here's an overview:

Causes:

- Bacterial Meningitis: Streptococcus pneumoniae and Neisseria meningitidis are common causes of bacterial meningitis in older adults.
- Viral Meningitis: Viral causes, such as herpes simplex virus (HSV) and

varicella-zoster virus (VZV), are also possible.

- Other Pathogens: Fungal and non-infectious causes are less common but can occur.

Risk Factors:

- Advanced Age: Older adults, especially those over 65, are at higher risk due to age-related changes in the immune system.
- Underlying Health Conditions: Chronic medical conditions, such as diabetes, heart disease, and immunosuppression, increase the risk.
- Close Contact: Living in communal settings, such as nursing homes, can increase the risk of exposure to pathogens.

Clinical Presentation:

- Symptoms can be subtle and nonspecific, including fever, altered mental status, confusion, headache, and neck stiffness.

- Older adults may present with atypical symptoms or may not exhibit classic signs of meningitis.

Diagnosis:

- Clinical Evaluation: A thorough history, physical exam, and assessment of mental status are crucial.
- Lumbar Puncture: A lumbar puncture is performed to collect cerebrospinal fluid (CSF) for analysis, which is essential for diagnosing meningitis.
- Blood Tests: Blood tests may be done to check for signs of infection and inflammation.

Treatment:

- Bacterial Meningitis: Prompt treatment with antibiotics is essential and may require hospitalization. The choice of antibiotics depends on the likely causative organism and local resistance patterns.

- Viral Meningitis: Treatment is generally supportive, as most cases of viral meningitis in older adults resolve on their own.
- Fungal Meningitis: Treatment with antifungal medications may be necessary for fungal causes.

Prevention:

- Vaccination: Vaccination against pneumococcus and meningococcus is recommended for older adults, as well as vaccination against influenza and other vaccine-preventable diseases.
- Hygiene: Practicing good hygiene, such as regular handwashing, can help prevent the spread of infections.

Meningitis in the elderly can be challenging to diagnose and manage due to atypical presentations and underlying health conditions. Early recognition, prompt treatment, and preventive measures are key to reducing the burden of meningitis in older adults.

8.3 Meningitis in Immunocompromised Individuals

Meningitis in immunocompromised individuals presents unique challenges due to the increased risk of severe and opportunistic infections. The causes, clinical presentation, diagnosis, and management differ from those in immunocompetent individuals. Here's an overview:

Causes:

- Bacterial Meningitis: Similar to immunocompetent individuals, bacterial causes such as Streptococcus pneumoniae, Neisseria meningitidis, and Listeria monocytogenes are common.

- Viral Meningitis: Viral causes, including herpes simplex virus (HSV), varicella-zoster virus (VZV), and cytomegalovirus (CMV), can be more common in immunocompromised individuals.
- Fungal and Other Pathogens: Opportunistic pathogens, such as Cryptococcus neoformans, Candida species, and Mycobacterium tuberculosis, are more likely to cause meningitis in immunocompromised individuals.

Risk Factors:

- Immunodeficiency: Conditions such as HIV/AIDS, organ transplantation, cancer (especially hematologic malignancies), and immunosuppressive therapy increase the risk.
- Age: Older age is a risk factor due to age-related changes in the immune system.

- Underlying Health Conditions: Chronic medical conditions and comorbidities can contribute to immunocompromise.

Clinical Presentation:

- Symptoms can be similar to those in immunocompetent individuals but may progress more rapidly and be more severe.
- Atypical presentations, such as absence of fever or neck stiffness, can occur, especially in those with impaired immune responses.

Diagnosis:

- Clinical Evaluation: A thorough history, physical exam, and assessment of immunocompromising conditions are crucial.
- Lumbar Puncture: A lumbar puncture is performed to collect CSF for analysis, which is essential for diagnosing meningitis.

- Blood Tests: Blood tests may be done to check for signs of infection, immunodeficiency, and inflammation.

Treatment:

- Bacterial Meningitis: Prompt treatment with antibiotics is essential and may require hospitalization. The choice of antibiotics depends on the likely causative organism and local resistance patterns.
- Viral Meningitis: Treatment is generally supportive, as most cases of viral meningitis in immunocompromised individuals resolve on their own. Antiviral therapy may be considered for specific viral causes.
- Fungal and Other Pathogens: Treatment with antifungal or other antimicrobial medications may be necessary for opportunistic pathogens.

Prevention:

- Vaccination: Vaccination against pneumococcus, meningococcus, and other vaccine-preventable diseases is important for immunocompromised individuals.
- Infection Control: Measures to prevent exposure to pathogens, such as avoiding contact with sick individuals and practicing good hygiene, are crucial.

Chapter 9

Complications of Meningitis

9.1 Neurological Complications

Meningitis, regardless of the age group affected, can lead to various neurological complications, some of which can be severe and long-lasting. These complications can arise due to the inflammation of the meninges and the brain tissue, as well as from the direct effects of the causative organism. Here are some common neurological complications associated with meningitis:

1. **Hydrocephalus:** Meningitis can obstruct the normal flow of cerebrospinal fluid (CSF) within the brain, leading to an accumulation of fluid and increased pressure in the brain (hydrocephalus).

2. **Brain Abscess:** In some cases, bacteria or fungi causing the meningitis can form pockets of infection within the brain tissue, known as brain abscesses. These can cause focal neurological deficits and require surgical drainage.

3. **Seizures:** Meningitis can irritate the brain tissue, leading to seizures. Seizures may occur during the acute phase of the illness or as a long-term complication.

4. **Cranial Nerve Dysfunction:** Inflammation of the meninges can affect the cranial nerves, leading to symptoms such as double vision, facial weakness, or difficulty swallowing.

5. **Cognitive Impairment:** Meningitis can cause cognitive deficits, including memory problems, difficulty concentrating, and impaired executive function.

6. **Sensorineural Hearing Loss:** Meningitis, particularly bacterial meningitis, can

damage the cochlea or auditory nerve, leading to permanent hearing loss.

7. **Gait Disturbances:** Some individuals may experience difficulties with balance and coordination, which can affect walking (gait).

8. **Behavioral and Psychiatric Changes:** Meningitis can cause changes in behavior, mood, and personality, which may persist after the acute phase of the illness.

9. **Developmental Delays:** Infants and young children who experience meningitis may have developmental delays, including delays in motor skills, language development, and social skills.

10. **Long-term Cognitive Impairment:** In severe cases, particularly in bacterial meningitis, individuals may experience long-term cognitive impairment, including learning difficulties and intellectual disability.

The risk of neurological complications can be reduced with prompt diagnosis and appropriate treatment of meningitis. However, some complications may still occur despite treatment. Rehabilitation and supportive care are important for individuals who experience neurological sequelae of meningitis to optimize their recovery and quality of life.

9.2 Systemic Complications

1. **Sepsis:** Meningitis can lead to a systemic infection known as sepsis, where the body's immune response to the infection causes widespread inflammation. Sepsis can lead to organ dysfunction and failure.
2. **Septic Shock:** In severe cases of sepsis, the body's response to the infection can lead to a drop in blood pressure and insufficient blood flow to vital organs, resulting in septic shock, a life-threatening condition.
3. **Disseminated Intravascular Coagulation (DIC):** Meningitis can

trigger a cascade of events that leads to abnormal blood clotting throughout the body, followed by excessive bleeding. DIC can lead to organ damage and failure.

4. **Respiratory Failure:** Severe meningitis can affect the respiratory center in the brain or lead to sepsis-induced lung injury, resulting in respiratory failure.

5. **Acute Kidney Injury:** Sepsis and the inflammatory response associated with meningitis can damage the kidneys, leading to acute kidney injury.

6. **Cardiovascular Complications:** Meningitis can affect the heart, leading to arrhythmias (irregular heartbeats), myocarditis (inflammation of the heart muscle), and pericarditis (inflammation of the sac surrounding the heart).

7. **Hepatic Dysfunction:** Meningitis-associated sepsis can affect liver function, leading to hepatic dysfunction.

8. **Adrenal Insufficiency:** Severe illness, including meningitis, can lead to adrenal insufficiency, where the adrenal glands do not produce enough cortisol, a hormone essential for managing stress and maintaining blood pressure.

9. **Metabolic Disturbances:** Meningitis can lead to electrolyte imbalances, hypoglycemia (low blood sugar), and metabolic acidosis.

10. **Hematologic Complications:** Meningitis can lead to abnormalities in the blood, such as thrombocytopenia (low platelet count) or leukopenia (low white blood cell count).

The systemic complications of meningitis highlight the importance of early diagnosis and aggressive treatment to prevent severe illness and improve outcomes. Management of systemic complications often involves intensive care and supportive measures tailored to the individual's specific needs.

9.3 Long-Term Sequelae

Meningitis can have long-term sequelae, particularly if not promptly diagnosed and treated. These sequelae can affect various aspects of health and quality of life. Here are some common long-term sequelae associated with meningitis:

1. **Neurological Deficits:** Meningitis can lead to lasting neurological problems, such as cognitive impairment, memory deficits, learning difficulties, and problems with concentration and attention.

2. **Hearing Loss:** Sensorineural hearing loss is a common long-term complication of bacterial meningitis, particularly in children. It can range from mild to profound and may require hearing aids or other interventions.

3. **Vision Problems:** Meningitis can lead to vision problems, including blindness, due to optic nerve damage or other ocular complications.

4. **Seizures:** Some individuals may develop epilepsy or recurrent seizures following meningitis.

5. **Motor Impairment:** Meningitis can cause weakness, paralysis, or coordination problems due to damage to the brain or spinal cord.

6. **Behavioral and Psychiatric Issues:** Meningitis survivors may experience behavioral changes, mood disorders, anxiety, depression, or post-traumatic stress disorder (PTSD).

7. **Developmental Delays:** Infants and young children who survive meningitis may experience delays in physical, cognitive, or social development.

8. **Chronic Fatigue:** Some individuals may experience long-lasting fatigue and

decreased energy levels following meningitis.

9. **Headaches:** Chronic headaches are a common complaint among meningitis survivors, which can significantly impact quality of life.

10. **Post-Meningitis Syndrome:** Some individuals may experience a constellation of symptoms known as post-meningitis syndrome, which can include headaches, fatigue, memory problems, and difficulty concentrating.

11. **Emotional and Social Impact:** Meningitis survivors may face emotional and social challenges due to the physical and cognitive sequelae of the illness.

The long-term sequelae of meningitis highlight the importance of early diagnosis, prompt treatment, and comprehensive rehabilitation and support services for survivors. Regular follow-up care is essential to monitor for and manage any long-term complications.

Chapter 10

Post-Meningitis Care and Rehabilitation

10.1 Monitoring and Follow-Up

Monitoring and follow-up care for individuals who have had meningitis are important to assess recovery, manage any ongoing symptoms or complications, and prevent future episodes. The specific monitoring and follow-up recommendations may vary depending on the individual's age, the underlying cause of meningitis, and the presence of any complications. Here are some key aspects of monitoring and follow-up care:

1. **Neurological Assessment:** Regular neurological examinations may be conducted to assess for any lingering

deficits or changes in neurological function.

2. **Hearing Tests:** Hearing assessments, such as audiograms, may be recommended, especially for individuals who had bacterial meningitis, to detect any hearing loss and determine the need for hearing aids or other interventions.

3. **Vision Screening:** Regular eye examinations may be recommended to monitor for any vision problems or changes in visual acuity.

4. **Cognitive Assessment:** Cognitive assessments may be performed to evaluate memory, attention, and other cognitive functions, especially in individuals who report ongoing cognitive difficulties.

5. **Psychological Evaluation:** Individuals experiencing emotional or psychological issues, such as anxiety, depression, or PTSD, may benefit from psychological evaluation and counseling.

6. **Vaccination:** Ensuring that individuals are up-to-date on recommended vaccinations, including those against pneumococcus, meningococcus, and influenza, is important to prevent future episodes of meningitis.

7. **Follow-Up Imaging:** In some cases, follow-up imaging studies, such as MRI or CT scans, may be recommended to assess for any structural changes in the brain or complications such as hydrocephalus or abscess formation.

8. **Medication Management:** Individuals who require long-term medication management, such as anticonvulsants for seizures or antibiotics for recurrent infections, may need regular follow-up with healthcare providers.

9. **Rehabilitation Services:** Some individuals may benefit from rehabilitation services, such as physical therapy, occupational therapy, or speech

therapy, to address any lingering physical or cognitive deficits.

10. **Education and Support:** Providing education and support to individuals and their families about the long-term effects of meningitis and strategies for managing ongoing symptoms or complications can be beneficial.

10.2 Rehabilitation Services

Rehabilitation services play a crucial role in the recovery and management of individuals who have had meningitis, especially those who experience lingering physical, cognitive, or emotional effects. Rehabilitation aims to improve functional abilities, enhance quality of life, and promote independence. Here are some key rehabilitation services that may be beneficial for individuals recovering from meningitis:

1. **Physical Therapy (PT):** Physical therapists can help individuals improve strength, flexibility, balance, and coordination. PT can also help manage muscle weakness, joint stiffness, and gait abnormalities that may result from meningitis.

2. **Occupational Therapy (OT):** Occupational therapists focus on improving activities of daily living (ADLs), such as dressing, feeding, and bathing. They also help individuals develop strategies to improve cognitive skills and manage fatigue.

3. **Speech Therapy:** Speech therapists work with individuals who experience speech and language difficulties following meningitis. They can help improve communication skills, swallowing function, and cognitive-communication skills.

4. **Cognitive Rehabilitation:** Cognitive rehabilitation programs are designed to

address memory, attention, and executive function deficits that may result from meningitis. These programs can include cognitive exercises, strategies for improving memory and attention, and education about brain health.

5. **Psychological Support:** Psychologists or counselors can provide support and counseling to individuals who experience emotional or psychological issues, such as anxiety, depression, or PTSD, following meningitis. They can also help individuals cope with any changes in their abilities or lifestyle.

6. **Vocational Rehabilitation:** Vocational rehabilitation services can help individuals return to work or school after meningitis. This may include vocational assessment, job training, and support in finding suitable employment or educational opportunities.

7. **Assistive Devices:** Rehabilitation specialists can assess the need for and

provide assistive devices, such as mobility aids, communication devices, or adaptive equipment, to help individuals function more independently.

8. **Home Modifications:** Occupational therapists can assess the home environment and recommend modifications or adaptations to improve safety and accessibility for individuals with physical or cognitive impairments.

9. **Community Reintegration:** Rehabilitation services can help individuals reintegrate into their communities and participate in social, recreational, and leisure activities that are meaningful to them.

10. **Education and Training:** Rehabilitation providers can educate individuals and their families about the effects of meningitis and provide training in self-care techniques, coping strategies, and injury prevention.

10.3 Support for Patients and Caregivers

1. **Healthcare Team:** The healthcare team, including doctors, nurses, therapists, and social workers, can provide information, guidance, and medical care throughout the recovery process.
2. **Support Groups:** Joining a support group for individuals recovering from meningitis or caregivers can provide a sense of community, shared experiences, and practical tips for coping.
3. **Counseling:** Individual or family counseling can help patients and caregivers address emotional issues, such as anxiety, depression, or stress, related to the illness.
4. **Education:** Learning about meningitis, its effects, and strategies for managing symptoms can empower patients and caregivers to take an active role in recovery.

5. **Respite Care:** Caregivers may benefit from respite care services, which provide temporary relief from caregiving responsibilities to prevent burnout.

6. **Financial Assistance:** Financial assistance programs or resources may be available to help with medical expenses, caregiving costs, or other financial burdens related to the illness.

7. **Legal and Advocacy Support:** Legal and advocacy organizations can provide guidance on legal rights, disability benefits, and advocacy efforts for individuals affected by meningitis.

8. **Community Services:** Community organizations, religious groups, or local charities may offer practical support, such as meal delivery, transportation assistance, or home visits.

9. **Online Resources:** Websites, forums, and online communities dedicated to meningitis can provide information,

support, and a platform for sharing experiences.

10. **Care Coordination:** Care coordination services can help patients and caregivers navigate the healthcare system, access resources, and coordinate care among various providers.

Chapter 11

Meningitis Outbreaks and Public Health

11.1 Surveillance and Reporting

1. **Case Definition:** Health authorities establish a case definition for meningitis, specifying criteria such as symptoms, laboratory results, and epidemiological factors that must be met for a case to be considered confirmed.

2. **Laboratory Testing:** Laboratory confirmation of meningitis cases is crucial. This often involves testing cerebrospinal fluid (CSF) obtained through a lumbar puncture to identify the causative organism (e.g., bacteria, virus, fungus).

3. **Healthcare Provider Reporting:** Healthcare providers are required to report suspected or confirmed cases of meningitis to local health authorities. This is typically done through electronic reporting systems or by phone.

4. **Laboratory Reporting:** Laboratories that perform testing for meningitis-causing pathogens report positive results to public health authorities, along with relevant patient information.

5. **Data Collection and Analysis:** Public health agencies collect and analyze reported data to monitor disease trends, identify clusters or outbreaks, and assess the impact of interventions.

6. **Outbreak Investigation:** When clusters or outbreaks of meningitis are identified, public health authorities conduct investigations to determine the source of the outbreak, implement control measures, and prevent further spread.

7. **Surveillance Systems:** Surveillance systems for meningitis vary by country and region but often include national or regional databases that collect and store information on reported cases.
8. **International Reporting:** Some countries participate in international reporting systems, such as the World Health Organization's (WHO) Global Invasive Bacterial Vaccine-Preventable Diseases (IBVPD) network, to share data on meningitis and other diseases.
9. **Vaccine Surveillance:** Surveillance of meningitis vaccine coverage and effectiveness is important for assessing the impact of vaccination programs and identifying areas where additional efforts are needed.
10. **Public Health Action:** Surveillance data inform public health actions, such as vaccination campaigns, public education efforts, and recommendations for healthcare providers.

11.2 Response Strategies

1. **Case Management:** Prompt diagnosis and treatment of meningitis cases are essential to prevent complications and reduce transmission. Healthcare providers should follow established treatment guidelines for bacterial, viral, or fungal meningitis.
2. **Contact Tracing:** Identifying and monitoring individuals who have been in close contact with confirmed cases can help prevent further transmission. Close contacts may be offered prophylactic treatment or vaccination, depending on the type of meningitis.
3. **Vaccination:** Vaccination is a key strategy for preventing meningitis, particularly for bacterial causes such as Neisseria meningitidis, Streptococcus pneumoniae, and Haemophilus influenzae type b (Hib). Vaccination campaigns may be conducted

in outbreak settings to boost immunity in the population.

4. **Chemoprophylaxis:** In certain situations, chemoprophylaxis (preventive treatment with antibiotics) may be recommended for close contacts of meningitis cases to reduce the risk of secondary cases.

5. **Public Education:** Public health agencies should provide information to the public about meningitis, its symptoms, and prevention strategies. This can help raise awareness and encourage early seeking of medical care.

6. **Enhanced Surveillance:** During an outbreak, surveillance efforts may be intensified to monitor disease trends, identify new cases, and assess the impact of control measures.

7. **Environmental Measures:** In healthcare settings, infection control measures such as hand hygiene, isolation precautions, and proper sterilization of medical

equipment can help prevent healthcare-associated infections.

8. **Outbreak Investigation:** Public health agencies conduct thorough investigations of meningitis outbreaks to determine the source, mode of transmission, and risk factors. This information guides control measures and prevention efforts.

9. **Capacity Building:** Strengthening healthcare infrastructure, laboratory capacity, and surveillance systems can improve the ability to detect, respond to, and control meningitis outbreaks.

10. **Research and Development:** Continued research into meningitis prevention, treatment, and vaccines is important for improving outcomes and reducing the burden of the disease.

11.3 Vaccination Programs

1. **Routine Childhood Vaccination:** Many countries include meningitis vaccines in their routine childhood vaccination schedules. Vaccines against Hib, pneumococcus, and meningococcus are commonly administered to infants and young children to protect against these bacterial causes of meningitis.

2. **Adolescent and College Vaccination:** Adolescents and college students are at higher risk of meningococcal meningitis due to social factors. Vaccination programs often target this age group, particularly before entry to college, to prevent outbreaks in crowded settings.

3. **Travel Vaccination:** Travelers to regions where meningitis is endemic or where outbreaks are occurring may be advised to receive meningitis vaccines, particularly against meningococcus serogroups A, C, W, and Y.

4. **Outbreak Response Vaccination:** During meningitis outbreaks, targeted vaccination campaigns may be conducted to vaccinate high-risk populations and prevent further transmission. These campaigns often involve mass vaccination efforts in affected communities.

5. **Vaccination for High-Risk Groups:** Individuals with certain medical conditions or risk factors, such as immunocompromised individuals or those with functional or anatomical asplenia, may be recommended to receive meningitis vaccines as part of their routine medical care.

6. **Vaccine Development and Introduction:** Continued research and development of new meningitis vaccines, including those targeting emerging serogroups or novel pathogens, are important for improving vaccine coverage and effectiveness.

7. **Vaccine Safety Monitoring:** Monitoring the safety of meningitis vaccines is

essential to detect and respond to any adverse events following immunization. Surveillance systems are in place to monitor vaccine safety and inform public health decision-making.

Chapter 12

Research and Future Directions

12.1 Current Research Trends

1. **Vaccine Development:** Researchers are working on developing new vaccines and improving existing vaccines for meningitis. This includes vaccines targeting emerging serogroups, such as meningococcus serogroup X, as well as vaccines with broader coverage against multiple serogroups.

2. **Genomic Studies:** Genomic studies are helping researchers better understand the genetic makeup of meningitis-causing pathogens, which can inform vaccine development and treatment strategies.

3. **Diagnostic Advances:** Advances in diagnostic techniques, such as molecular testing and rapid point-of-care tests, are improving the speed and accuracy of meningitis diagnosis, particularly in resource-limited settings.

4. **Immune Response Studies:** Studying the immune response to meningitis is providing insights into how the body responds to infection and how vaccines can stimulate protective immunity.

5. **Antimicrobial Resistance:** Researchers are studying antimicrobial resistance patterns in meningitis-causing pathogens to inform treatment guidelines and strategies for preventing the spread of resistant strains.

6. **Host-Pathogen Interactions:** Understanding the interactions between the host and the pathogen is helping researchers develop new therapeutic approaches that target specific pathways involved in infection and inflammation.

7. **Neurological Complications:** Research is focused on identifying risk factors for neurological complications following meningitis and developing interventions to prevent or reduce long-term sequelae.

8. **Epidemiological Studies:** Epidemiological studies are helping researchers understand the global burden of meningitis, identify high-risk populations, and guide vaccination strategies.

9. **Clinical Trials:** Clinical trials are evaluating new treatments, vaccine candidates, and diagnostic tools for meningitis to determine their safety and efficacy in real-world settings.

10. **Public Health Interventions:** Research is informing public health interventions, such as vaccination campaigns and outbreak response strategies, to control and prevent meningitis outbreaks.

12.2 Emerging Therapies and Vaccines

1. **Novel Vaccines:** Researchers are developing new vaccines to target additional serogroups of meningococcus, such as serogroup B, which has been challenging to vaccinate against due to its unique structure. These vaccines aim to provide broader coverage against multiple serogroups.

2. **Conjugate Vaccines:** Conjugate vaccines are being developed to improve the immune response and effectiveness of existing vaccines against meningococcus, pneumococcus, and Hib. These vaccines link the bacterial polysaccharide to a carrier protein to enhance the immune response.

3. **Multivalent Vaccines:** Multivalent vaccines are being developed to provide protection against multiple serogroups or strains of meningitis-causing pathogens in

a single vaccine formulation. This approach can simplify vaccination schedules and improve coverage.

4. **Pneumococcal Vaccines:** New pneumococcal vaccines are being developed to target additional strains of Streptococcus pneumoniae, which is a leading cause of bacterial meningitis. These vaccines aim to provide broader protection against pneumococcal disease.

5. **Therapeutic Vaccines:** Therapeutic vaccines are being investigated as a potential treatment for meningitis. These vaccines stimulate the immune system to target and eliminate pathogens already present in the body, potentially reducing the severity and duration of infection.

6. **Immunomodulators:** Immunomodulatory therapies are being studied to modulate the immune response in meningitis, potentially reducing inflammation and tissue damage. These

therapies aim to improve outcomes and reduce the risk of long-term sequelae.

7. **Antimicrobial Therapies:** Researchers are exploring new antimicrobial agents and treatment regimens for meningitis, particularly in cases of antimicrobial resistance. These therapies aim to improve treatment outcomes and reduce the risk of treatment failure.

8. **Host-Directed Therapies:** Host-directed therapies are being investigated to target host pathways involved in the immune response to meningitis. These therapies aim to modulate the host response to infection, potentially improving outcomes and reducing tissue damage.

9. **Nanotechnology-Based Therapies:** Nanotechnology-based therapies are being developed to deliver antimicrobial agents or vaccines more effectively to target tissues in the central nervous system, potentially improving treatment outcomes and reducing side effects.

10. **Gene Therapies:** Gene therapies are being explored as a potential treatment for meningitis, aiming to modify the genetic makeup of host cells to enhance the immune response or target specific pathogens.

12.3 Challenges and Opportunities

Challenges:

1. **Antimicrobial Resistance:** The emergence of antimicrobial-resistant strains of bacteria, such as Neisseria meningitidis and Streptococcus pneumoniae, poses a challenge for the treatment of meningitis.

2. **Vaccine Coverage and Access:** Ensuring high vaccination coverage, especially in low- and middle-income countries,

remains a challenge. Access to vaccines, particularly in remote or underserved areas, is also a concern.

3. **Diagnostic Delays:** Delays in the diagnosis of meningitis can lead to delayed treatment and poor outcomes. Improving access to rapid diagnostic tests and laboratory facilities is important.

4. **Emerging Pathogens:** The identification of new pathogens causing meningitis, as well as changes in the epidemiology of existing pathogens, presents challenges for prevention and treatment strategies.

5. **Neurological Sequelae:** Long-term neurological sequelae, such as cognitive impairment, hearing loss, and motor deficits, can occur in survivors of meningitis, highlighting the need for comprehensive rehabilitation services.

6. **Public Awareness:** Lack of public awareness about meningitis, its symptoms, and prevention measures can lead to

delays in seeking medical care and contribute to the spread of the disease.

7. **Vaccine Hesitancy:** Vaccine hesitancy, fueled by misinformation and mistrust, can hinder vaccination efforts and increase the risk of outbreaks.

8. **Healthcare Infrastructure:** Inadequate healthcare infrastructure, particularly in resource-limited settings, can limit access to timely diagnosis and treatment of meningitis.

Opportunities:

1. **Advancements in Vaccines:** Advances in vaccine development, including new conjugate vaccines and multivalent vaccines, offer opportunities to improve coverage and protection against meningitis-causing pathogens.

2. **Technological Innovations:** Technological innovations, such as rapid diagnostic tests, telemedicine, and mobile health applications, can improve access to

timely diagnosis and treatment of meningitis, especially in remote or underserved areas.

3. **Global Collaboration:** Collaboration among researchers, healthcare providers, governments, and international organizations can facilitate the sharing of knowledge, resources, and best practices for meningitis prevention and control.

4. **Research and Development:** Continued research into the pathogenesis of meningitis, host-pathogen interactions, and novel treatment strategies can lead to innovative approaches for prevention and treatment.

5. **Public Health Interventions:** Public health interventions, such as vaccination campaigns, surveillance programs, and outbreak response strategies, are key to controlling meningitis outbreaks and reducing the burden of the disease.

6. **Education and Awareness:** Education and awareness campaigns can help

improve knowledge about meningitis and promote vaccination and early medical care-seeking behaviors.

7. **Health System Strengthening:** Strengthening healthcare systems, particularly in low- and middle-income countries, can improve access to quality care for individuals affected by meningitis.

Chapter 13

Conclusion

13.1 Recap of Key Points

1. **Definition:** Meningitis is the inflammation of the meninges, the protective membranes covering the brain and spinal cord, usually caused by infection.
2. **Types:** Meningitis can be classified into several types based on the cause:
   - Bacterial Meningitis: Caused by bacteria such as Neisseria meningitidis, Streptococcus pneumoniae, and Haemophilus influenzae.
   - Viral Meningitis: Caused by viruses, with enteroviruses being the most common.

- o Fungal Meningitis: Caused by fungi such as Cryptococcus neoformans.
  - o Parasitic Meningitis: Caused by parasites such as Naegleria fowleri and Trypanosoma brucei.

3. **Epidemiology:** Meningitis can occur at any age but is more common in infants, children, adolescents, and the elderly. Certain factors, such as travel, living in crowded settings, and immunocompromised status, can increase the risk.

4. **Transmission:** Meningitis is usually transmitted through respiratory droplets, direct contact with an infected person, or ingestion of contaminated food or water.

5. **Clinical Features:** Symptoms of meningitis can include fever, headache, neck stiffness, photophobia (sensitivity to light), and altered mental status. In infants, symptoms may also include irritability, poor feeding, and a bulging fontanelle.

6. **Diagnosis:** Diagnosis is based on clinical evaluation, imaging studies (such as CT or MRI scans), and analysis of cerebrospinal fluid (CSF) obtained through a lumbar puncture.

7. **Treatment:** Treatment depends on the type and cause of meningitis but often includes antibiotics or antiviral medications. Supportive care to manage symptoms and complications is also important.

8. **Prevention:** Prevention strategies include vaccination, good hygiene practices (such as handwashing), and avoiding close contact with infected individuals.

9. **Complications:** Meningitis can lead to various complications, including neurological deficits, hearing loss, and cognitive impairment. Prompt diagnosis and treatment are crucial to prevent these complications.

10. **Emerging Therapies and Vaccines:** Researchers are developing new vaccines

and therapies for meningitis, including novel vaccines targeting additional serogroups and antimicrobial therapies.

11. **Challenges and Opportunities:** Challenges include antimicrobial resistance, vaccine coverage gaps, and diagnostic delays, while opportunities include advancements in vaccines, technological innovations, and global collaboration.

12. **Monitoring and Response:** Surveillance and reporting of meningitis cases are essential for monitoring disease trends, identifying outbreaks, and guiding public health interventions. Response strategies include case management, contact tracing, vaccination campaigns, and public education efforts.

13.2 Importance of Early Detection and Treatment

1. **Prevention of Complications:** Prompt treatment can prevent serious complications such as brain damage, hearing loss, and cognitive impairment. It can also reduce the risk of death, especially in bacterial meningitis.
2. **Reduction of Spread:** Early detection and treatment can help prevent the spread of meningitis to others, especially in cases where the infection is contagious. This is important for preventing outbreaks in communities and healthcare settings.
3. **Improved Outcomes:** Early treatment is associated with better outcomes, including shorter illness duration, less severe symptoms, and improved overall recovery.
4. **Symptom Management:** Early treatment can help manage symptoms such as fever, headache, and neck stiffness, improving

the patient's comfort and quality of life during the illness.

5. **Prevention of Long-Term Effects:** Some individuals may experience long-term neurological or cognitive effects following meningitis. Early treatment can reduce the risk of these effects and improve long-term outcomes.

6. **Avoidance of Unnecessary Tests:** Early diagnosis can help avoid unnecessary tests and interventions, as healthcare providers can quickly confirm the presence of meningitis and start appropriate treatment.

7. **Guidance for Public Health Measures:** Early detection of meningitis cases allows public health authorities to implement timely control measures, such as contact tracing and vaccination campaigns, to prevent further spread.

13.3 Hope for the Future

There is hope for the future in the fight against meningitis, thanks to ongoing research, advances in technology, and global collaboration. Here are some reasons to be hopeful:

1. **Advancements in Vaccines:** Researchers are making significant progress in developing new vaccines and improving existing ones for meningitis. These vaccines have the potential to provide broader coverage, longer-lasting immunity, and better protection against emerging strains.

2. **Improved Diagnostic Tools:** Advances in diagnostic techniques, such as rapid molecular tests and point-of-care devices, are making it easier to quickly and accurately diagnose meningitis. This can lead to faster treatment and better outcomes.

3. **Enhanced Surveillance Systems:** Improvements in surveillance systems

allow for better monitoring of meningitis trends, early detection of outbreaks, and more targeted public health interventions.

4. **Technological Innovations:** Technologies such as telemedicine, mobile health apps, and digital health records are improving access to healthcare services, especially in remote or underserved areas, and facilitating timely diagnosis and treatment of meningitis.

5. **Global Collaboration:** Collaboration among researchers, healthcare providers, governments, and international organizations is helping to share knowledge, resources, and best practices for meningitis prevention and control.

6. **Increased Awareness:** Public awareness campaigns are raising awareness about meningitis, its symptoms, and the importance of vaccination and early treatment. This can lead to earlier detection and improved outcomes for individuals affected by the disease.

7. **Health System Strengthening:** Efforts to strengthen healthcare systems, particularly in low- and middle-income countries, are improving access to quality care for individuals with meningitis and other infectious diseases.

8. **Research and Development:** Ongoing research into the pathogenesis of meningitis, host-pathogen interactions, and novel treatment strategies is expanding our understanding of the disease and paving the way for new and more effective treatments.